Cheap & Effective Home Remedies
Cures to help treat the top 20 most common conditions

Innana Canon
© Copyright 2016

I0440515

Table of Contents

Disclaimer 3

Introduction 3

1-Hypertension 4

2-Hyperlipidemia (elevated cholesterol) 7

3-Diabetes 10

4-Arthritis 13

5-Anxiety 16

6-Asthma 19

7-Hypothyroidism 22

8-Cellulite 24

9-Multiple Sclerosis 27

10-Urinary Tract Infection (UTI) 31

11-Constipation 35

12-Greying hair 38

13-Eczema 39

14-Erectile Dysfunction & Impotence 42

15-Dandruff 44

16-Migraine Headaches 46

.... 46

17-Breast Cancer 48

18-Ovarian Cysts 50

19-Brittle Nails 53

20-Irritable Bowel Syndrome (IBS) 55

Conclusion: 57

Disclaimer

The information provided within this eBook is for general informational purposes only. While the Author tries to keep the information up-to-date and correct, there are no representations or warranties, expressed or implied, about the completeness, accuracy, reliability, suitability or availability with respect to the information, products, services, or related graphics contained in this eBook for any purpose. Any use of this information is at your own risk.

This eBook contains information that is intended to help the readers be better informed on possible natural home remedies. It is presented as general advice on the subject. Always consult your doctor for your individual needs.

This book is not intended to be a substitute for the medical advice of a licensed physician. The reader should consult with their doctor in any matters relating to his/her health.

Introduction

Thank you for downloading this eBook! My hope is that the information contained within these pages brings you hope, relief, and healing. By nature, our bodies are designed to move away from disease and move towards health. Nature makes no mistakes and a remedy for your disease does exist naturally!

Let's face it, we don't need pharmaceuticals to be healthy. When given the proper nutritional support, the body can heal itself without the need for toxic and expensive medicine. That's not to say that all conventional medicine is without value but rather that there are alternative remedies that should be explored first and for long enough to give the body a fighting chance.

In this guide, I have selected some of my favorite remedies for common conditions that most Americans have suffered or know someone who has suffered with. These cures are practical and affordable and more than likely, contain items that can easily be picked up from a grocery or local health food store.

1-Hypertension

As being one of the most common conditions affecting both men and women, hypertension or high blood pressure is said to affect more than 70 million American adults and that number is rapidly growing. Typical medical treatments for this condition include prescription medication such as beta-blockers and ACE inhibitor drugs both of which are dangerous and with prolonged use, can lead to problems in other areas of the body. Although these drugs are effective in treating the condition, they do not address the underlying problem.

In addition to prescribing drugs, Doctors urge patients to limit the amount salt in their diet. This has been one of the biggest theories in relation to hypertension yet there just is not enough evidence to prove it. In fact, numerous studies have proven time after time that a salt restricted diet does not help to cure hypertension.

So what is the best remedy for high blood pressure?

Calcium and lots of it! Foods high in calcium may help but must be used in conjunction with supplements. Also, in order for calcium to work effectively, adding vitamin D and Magnesium can help.

Numerous theories conclude that calcium helps to keep the body alkaline by preventing the body's pH level from becoming acidic. This works because hypertension cannot be prevalent in an alkaline body.

What other natural cures can you use for hypertension?

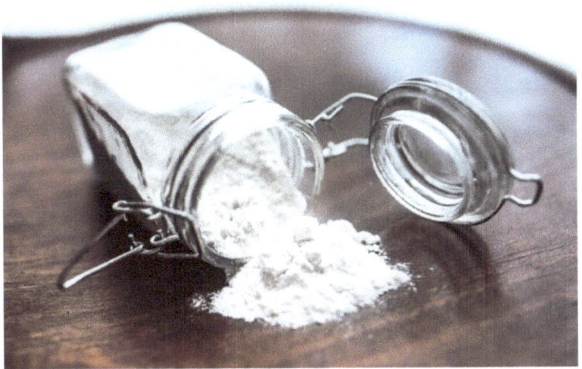

Baking Soda. Yes, you read that correctly. Baking soda is easily one of the fastest most affordable ways to lower hypertension naturally. Best of all, you probably already have a box laying around somewhere in your pantry since it is such a common kitchen item.

Baking soda is an excellent way to boost your pH levels quickly and efficiently. It's important to monitor your body's pH levels regularly to ensure that this method is working for you and to help measure the difference. An easy way to do this is to pick up alkaline test strips which can detect and measure the body's pH levels through urine.

How to take:

Mix 1/8 teaspoon of baking soda in 1 cup of water and add 2 tbsp. of apple cider vinegar and take twice daily. This should be repeated for approximately two weeks. After that, take only the apple cider vinegar and water alone for another two weeks. Once the two weeks are up, you may resume adding the baking soda. Continue this two weeks on and off cycle with the baking soda until you begin to see an improvement in your symptoms.

Since this is a safe and natural method, it can be continued for as long as you wish as long as you follow the directions above.

Potassium which is found in a number of common foods is known to essentially "clean out" artery walls and flush excess sodium from the body. One of the best sources of potassium is liquid organic or unpasteurized apple cider vinegar which contains beneficial microorganisms and enzymes also known as the "Mother" apple.

2-Hyperlipidemia (elevated cholesterol)

If your recent blood work showed that you have elevated cholesterol and triglyceride levels, chances are, there is an underlying problem that needs addressing first. Taking cholesterol lowering drugs will only serve to treat the symptom but will not help to fix the cause of the problem.

There are a few common myths surrounding cholesterol that are pushed on the general public by health care providers and the pharmaceutical industry.

First Myth: The lower the cholesterol is in your body, the healthier you are. This could not be further from the truth. Cholesterol is essential to your health and overall well-being. In fact, the only time it becomes problematic is when there is an excess of it. Simply put, we cannot live without cholesterol. The "safe range" for this essential nutrient was once thought to be around 400 (4.0). Today, the "safe range" is below 200 (2.0). Despite this, death from heart disease has actually increased dramatically in the last 30 years and is expected to increase in years to come.

You're probably thinking, how does this make sense?

Cholesterol is crucial to the proper functioning of the nervous system and liver as well as a crucial building block for adrenal and sex hormones. What's more, only 10% of one's daily need comes from the human body. The rest must be supplied through ones diet.

Second Myth: Animal products high in cholesterol such as full fat milk products, eggs, and red meat, are bad for you. This theory has never been proven and in fact, numerous studies have disproven its credibility.

An Eskimos diet consists of 70% animal fat, meat, and cholesterol. Despite this, a research study conducted on Eskimo health proved that their cholesterol and triglyceride levels were found to be low and that their risks for heart disease, stroke, and cancer were even lower.

As far as eggs go, study after study has shown that eggs do not raise cholesterol levels. In fact, they have been said to lower cholesterol since they contain lecithin (which is known to naturally reduce cholesterol). So, let's through this myth out once and for all!

What about butter? This is another horrid myth perpetuated by the pharmaceutical industry. It appears that the real culprit is processed oils and margarine. Butter in and of itself is not proven to raise cholesterol. In fact, countries like Sweden and Denmark who are the biggest consumers of butter have shown to have normal cholesterol levels. So go ahead and spread some on your toast today!

Third Myth: High cholesterol is a disease caused by heredity. Ladies and gentleman, this is a pure theory that has never been proven to be true. Do not fall for this.

High cholesterol is caused primarily by an individual's diet and standard of living such as excessive alcohol consumption, smoking, nutrient imbalance, and having a sedentary lifestyle.

Now that we've discussed the myths, let's discuss what you can do if you have been diagnosed with high cholesterol

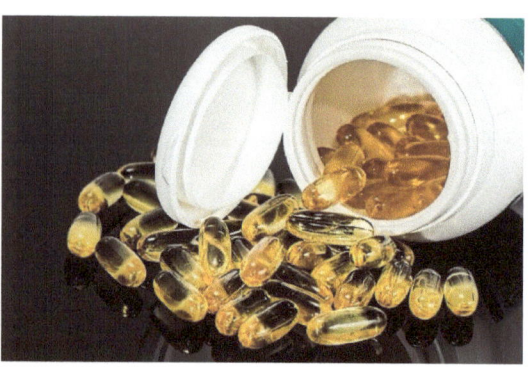

Fish oil supplement: I know, this one is pushed on us a lot...but there is a lot of evidence to back it up. Fish oil has been proven time after time to lower cholesterol and triglyceride levels. Consuming dark meat/cold water fish on a frequent basis can be just what you need. However, if you're not a big fan of fish, taking a good quality Omega-3 Supplement can be comparable.

Foods to incorporate into your diet to naturally lower cholesterol:

- **Oats:** bring triglyceride levels down fast due to the fiber it contains.

- **Apples:** Opt for organic apples whenever possible—any kind will do.
- **Avocados**: contain healthy mono-saturated fats, including oleic acid which has been shown to lower cholesterol.
- **Dark greens:** Spinach, broccoli, and lettuce to be specific. Try organic whenever possible.
- **Lecithin:** This can be purchased in supplemental form or is found in egg yolks.
- **Blueberries:** containing powerful antioxidants, bioflavonoids, and vitamin C, these little gems play a huge role in disease prevention overall.
- **Soy:** Aim for organic whenever possible. Soy will help to activate enzymes within the body to help reduce cholesterol.
- **Flax Seeds:** these can be added to a smoothie or sprinkled on your salad or cereal.
- **Garlic:** Helps to enhance the immune system and lower cholesterol and blood pressure levels.
- **Water:** aim for at least 2 liters of water per day for optimal results.

3-Diabetes

Over the last 10 years alone, the number of people diagnosed with diabetes has skyrocketed. It is now estimated that 25.8 million adults and children have this nasty disease. Left untreated, diabetes can potentially lead to a wide range of health risks including coma and death.

So what causes diabetes and what are some of the symptoms associated with it?

Normally, the body's metabolic process consists of converting carbohydrates into a sugar called glucose. This then circulates in a person's bloodstream and signals the pancreas to secrete a hormone called insulin. This is the hormone that initiates the body's cells to absorb the glucose.

Once the glucose is absorbed by the cell, it becomes fuel to help generate energy or gets stored as fat in the body. In a person who has diabetes, this delicate process is disrupted. Instead, the pancreas releases little to no insulin or the body's cells reject the insulin. This causes the cells to be starved of glucose leading to a wide variety of symptoms such as weakness, fatigue, and frequent urination. Symptoms range from mild to more severe symptoms such as labored breathing, trembling, dizziness, and in worst cases, loss of consciousness.

There are 2 types of diabetes mellitus and they are type I and type II. Type I develops in childhood years due to minimal or no insulin production by the pancreas. Type I diabetics are required to take synthetic insulin to help keep their glucose levels lowered.

Type II diabetes which is also known as adult-onsite diabetes is the most common making up 90-95% of all diabetics. In the case of type II diabetes, the pancreas over-produces insulin but it is not absorbed by the cells so it is left to circulate in the bloodstream until it is flushed out in urine. Constantly elevated levels of blood glucose poses serious health risks.

So, what can you do about Diabetes?

Besides exercising regularly and eating fresh organic fruits and veggies, there are a few different natural remedies you can try at home to help manage and eventually eliminate diabetes. Please keep in mind that you should never stop taking your diabetes medication or insulin without consulting with your doctor first. You should continue to monitor your insulin regularly until a plan of action has been established and started under the guidance of your health care provider.

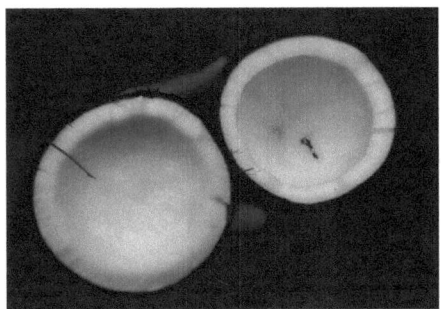

Coconut Oil. Yum! This miracle food has been known to treat a wide variety of illnesses and diabetes is definitely one of them. Best of all, it tastes great too. By consuming at least 3-4 tbsp. of coconut oil per day, you can successfully treat and reverse type II diabetes.

Coconut oil helps to reduce the constant sugar and carbohydrate cravings in individuals with diabetes. This helps to better control the body's blood sugar levels and keep them within normal range. Also, since most diabetics are also overweight, the coconut oil can also help with weight loss which in turn can help to manage diabetes better.

Black seeds: Nature's wonder seeds! Black seeds are an anti-inflammatory and immune system booster treating a score of illnesses which includes diabetes. A recent study showed that just 2 grams of black seeds a day helped to reduce fasting glucose levels, decrease insulin resistance, and increase cell function in diabetic participants.

The easiest way to take black seeds is to purchase the oil which can be found online or at most health food stores. For dosage information, refer to the directions contained on the bottle.

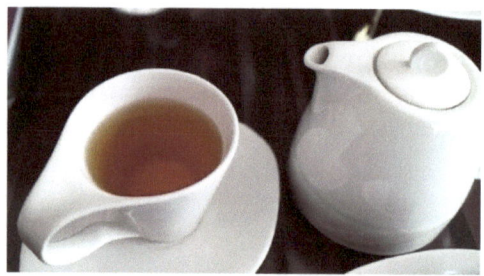

Green Tea can also be used to treat diabetes. It contains powerful polyphenol antioxidants which are well-known for increasing insulin sensitivity and stabilizing blood glucose levels.

Be sure to drink 4-6 cups a day for diabetes. Green tea supplements can be used instead if you cannot stomach the bitterness from the tea.

4-Arthritis

There are many natural remedies for arthritis that modern medical doctors fail to address. Unfortunately, this incredibility debilitating disease continues to affect millions of people worldwide.

Besides not being able to do the things they once were able to do, arthritis sufferers and their loved ones are severely misinformed about the types of natural treatments that are available to them. Most conventional medical treatments only focus on treating the symptoms of arthritis and fail to address the underlying problem.

Arthritis is an extremely profitable disease and the pharmaceutical industry is not interested in educating the masses on non-conventional treatments. Drug induced therapy appears to be the number one standard medical treatment available to patients for treating their arthritis. In the long run however, most of these medications are further damaging joints and overall health.

What's more, these drugs begin to lose their effectiveness over time requiring the need to switch medication and or increase the dosage. In addition, the medication can increase the risk for various illnesses such as heart attack, liver and kidney malfunction, and hypertension. The side effects associated with these medications can include depression, insomnia, and mood swings to name a few.

In addition to medication, surgery is oftentimes suggested by doctors to treat arthritis however this is a risky procedure that can cause serious complications.

So what can be done?

Baking soda and apple cider vinegar...yes again! This powerful combination is one of the most incredible ways to remedy arthritis naturally. I have tried this one personally and can vouch for it 100% (at least for me).

I mentioned some of the benefits of baking soda earlier but to recap, baking soda helps to elevate your body's pH levels. This helps to alkalize the body and keep it in a healthy state and since disease cannot live in an alkalized body, you should start to see relief immediately. It's crucial to keep in mind that you should not consume more than 2 tsp of baking soda a day to stay within the safe zone.

Apple cider vinegar is truly a powerful natural antibiotic which helps to heal the gut and destroy pathogens. In addition, it helps to replenish the digestive track with probiotics so that no bad bacteria can mess with your internal system! Pretty great if you ask me.

How to make remedy

Mix 2 tbsps. of apple cider vinegar with ½ teaspoon of baking soda in 1 cup of water. Add a teaspoon of black strap molasses or honey for extra benefit and taste. Drink twice daily and then gradually increase to three times daily. This can be done for 3 weeks and then the baking soda can be discontinued. You can continue to drink apple cider vinegar daily for as long as you want after that.

What else?

Turmeric & Ginger Tea. Both of these amazing ingredients are powerful anti-inflammatories which will help with the pain and swelling associated with arthritis. Turmeric contains a strong antioxidant that helps to lower the levels of two enzymes that are responsible for causing inflammation.

Here's how to take:

Combine 2 cups of water with a 1 teaspoon of ground turmeric, 1 teaspoon of ground ginger, and add honey to sweeten. Boil 2 cups of water and add the turmeric and ginger. Let simmer and then stand for 10 minutes. Finally, go ahead and strain it, add honey and enjoy! This can be enjoyed twice a day for as long as you'd like or until the pain is gone.

Blackstrap Molasses is a black syrup substance which is a by-product made by through the refining of sugar beets or sugarcane into sugar using a boiling process. Unlike regular sugar, molasses is rich in vitamins and minerals such as magnesium, calcium and potassium making it a potent home remedy for arthritis. Due to the nutrients contained within it, molasses helps to regulate the function of muscles and nerves and helps to make bones stronger.

Here's how to take:

This one is easy. Heat one cup of water until warm (not hot). Add 1 tbsp. of blackstrap molasses stir until dissolved. Drink one cup daily.

5-Anxiety

Anxiety and stress are unfortunately rampant in our society today and we all experience them on occasion. Anxiety is a natural response to stress or fear which alerts us to a perceived danger or threat. Without it, human beings would have no way of anticipating and adequately preparing for, an adverse situation ahead of them.

Anxiety only becomes problematic if it begins to affect ones daily life. This can easily spiral into a condition called Generalized Anxiety Disorder which is characterized by marked excessive worry regarding ordinary things. If you are like the millions of people around the world who suffer with this, understand that there are many natural remedies available for treatment.

Since anxiety produces many distressing physical symptoms such as a pounding heart, sweating, dizziness, and shortness of breath, it can cause added worry associated with the fear of death. The secret to treating these physical symptoms is to first calm the body and mind. A calm body will always lead to a calm mind and vice versa.

The good news is that there are many different home remedies you can use to alleviate anxiety and help calm your body down.

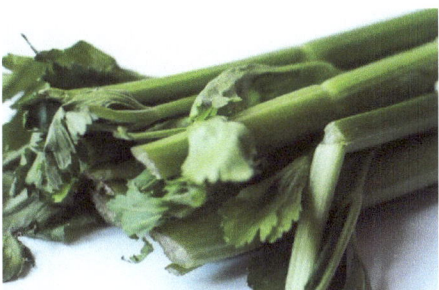

Celery. Stay with me now...Celery is high in folic acid and potassium. Deficiencies with either of these can cause nervousness. Consume approximately 2 cups of celery either raw or cooked with your meals for 2 weeks or until symptoms begin to subside.

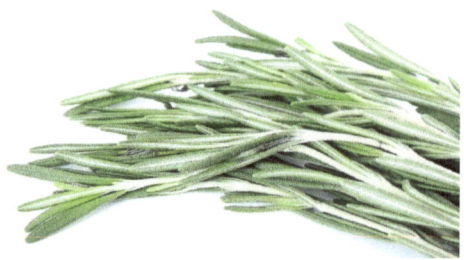

Rosemary: This popular spice has a calming effect on the nerves simply by inhaling the aroma. To enhance the benefits, burn a sprig or purchase rosemary oil and simply breathe in the aroma.

A tea can also be made from Rosemary to help ward off anxiety but adding 2 teaspoons of dried rosemary to 1 cup of boiling water. Let stand for 10 minutes and then drink.

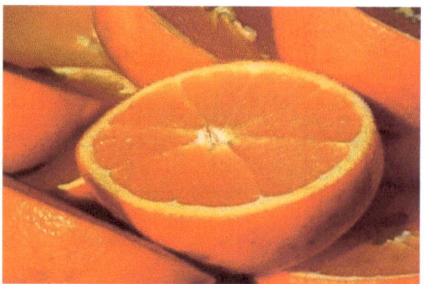

Orange. Who doesn't love a nice tall glass of OJ with their breakfast in the morning? Did you know it can also help with anxiety-induced tachycardia (racing heart). Simply mix 1 teaspoon of honey and a pinch of nutmeg into 1 cup of orange juice and drink.

Also, like the rosemary mentioned above, the aroma of orange has been known to reduce anxiety and its symptoms. You can inhale orange by simply peeling a fresh orange or boiling orange peels and simply breathing in the steam.

6-Asthma

Asthma is a chronic illness which involves the airways in the lungs which are responsible for allowing air to flow in and out of the lungs. Asthma occurs when this delicate process is disrupted due to inflammation of the airways causing the muscles around the airways to tighten making it difficult to breathe. Symptoms associated with is condition include shortness of breath, tightness in chest, coughing, and wheezing.

Over the last few years alone, reported cases of asthma have risen dramatically. It is now estimated that today, close to 34 million Americans have been diagnosed with asthma. In addition, according to the CDC, asthma costs upwards of 56 million dollars a year in medical costs, lost school and work days, and early deaths and this number is continuing to grow.

So what is the cause of this rampant growth of cases?

The theory that asthma is genetically inherited is just that, a theory! Therefore, there are other causes responsible for the incredible spike in asthma rates. Here are a few:

- **Increase in pollutants** which is found in our air, water, and food. Unfortunately, there is no way to eliminate these pollutants entirely but you can limit your exposure by cutting down on chemicals from the diet.
- **Decreased immunity in children and adults:** This should go without saying but when your immune system is compromised, your risks of contracting illnesses such as asthma increases. Therefore, you need to address the underlying problem by making sure you're taking care of your immune system.
- **Increased use of asthma medications:** Regular use of these medications can lead to an exacerbation in symptoms. This is because they negatively affect the immune system by causing a disruption to the body's endocrine system.

Is there anything you can do besides taking dangerous medication? Of course!

Hydrogren Peroxide Inhalation Therapy can be a very powerful natural remedy for asthma. Most people have this sitting in their medicine cabinet at home making it a very practical and affordable treatment. Best of all, it can work within minutes.

Here's the method:

1. Start by purchasing 3% food grade Hydrogren Peroxide and a nasal pump containing a generic nasal decongestant (you'll be dumping it out so the cheaper the better)
2. After emptying out the contents of the pump, make sure to sterilize the bottle properly using hot water and soap making sure all soap is properly rinsed out.
3. Fill the empty bottle with the peroxide and while pointing at the back of the throat, inhale and pump the spray 5-6 times (while inhaling). **Make sure that you are NOT inhaling it up the nose.

This method can be repeated 5 times a day or every 3 hours or so and can be used for as long as needed.

Another great home remedy is, **Ginger.** Due to it's anti-inflammatory components, this is actually one of the most effective herbs for helping to treat asthma symptoms. Ginger helps to relax and smoothen muscle tissue in the airways and can help to dissolve phlegm. Not to mention, it's excellent at boosting the immune system due to the powerful vitamins and minerals contained within it.

How to take?

The best way to enjoy ginger is by pouring boiling hot water on a few slices of ginger and letting it steep for 20 minutes before sipping. Add honey if desired. This can be enjoyed 2-3 times per day for as long as you'd like or until symptoms have decreased.

Home relief for asthma can also be achieved through consuming **garlic**. World renowned for its antiviral properties, garlic is an excellent anti-inflammatory food item that can be used for asthma. Garlic can easily be classified as "nature's antibiotic" as it can clear congestion in the nose, throat, and lungs and help to fight infections that typically trigger asthma attacks. Simply eat 1-2 cloves a day or use a garlic capsule to gain the most benefits.

7-Hypothyroidism

Hypothyroidism is the term that is used to describe an underactive thyroid gland. This is when the thyroid gland cannot keep up with normal hormone production to keep the body running normally. Common causes associated with this condition are autoimmune disease, radiation treatment, and the surgical removal of the thyroid.

Luckily, this condition is very easy to cure using simple remedies and treatments. Although there isn't a single cure that exists for hypothyroidism, relief can take place after an individual has modified his/her lifestyle and has incorporated vital supplements.

Traditional methods of treating hypothyroidism include modern day medicine and hormone therapy. Both of these methods can be harmful and even fatal especially when used in the long term.

Luckily, there are safer, more effective ways to treat this condition. Most of which the pharmaceutical industries will try and refute since it means zero profit for them. One way is to incorporate a healthy, well-balanced diet free from chemicals and processed sugar and rich in fruits, vegetables, and whole grains. In addition, it is also important to begin exercising on a frequent basis—even if it means just walking, get up and get moving.

Let's look at a few additional home remedies to try for hypothyroidism.

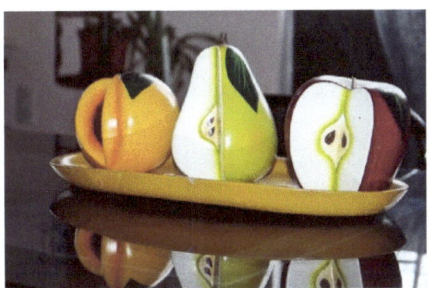

Apples, Pears, and Peaches. All are an excellent source of fiber which helps to keep you regular. This in turn helps to regulate hormones as well! All three of these fruits help to calm hormone imbalances in a woman's body helping her relax. They work best when combined.

Here is a wonderful juice recipe to try:

Combine 1-apple, 1-pear, and 2-peaches. Blend together and pour through a strainer to remove pulp if needed. This can be drank once daily for as long as you'd like or until signs and symptoms subside.

Vitamin D: This is best when derived from natural sunlight. It's important to get at least 30-minutes of natural sunlight exposure daily. Put away the sunblock and sunglasses during that time and really allow the sun to penetrate your skin and eyes. Allowing the sunlight to be absorbed adequately, helps to stimulate the body's pineal and pituitary glands. These glands are responsible for releasing T3 & R4 hormones which helps to speed up the body's metabolism. This can help lead to weight loss and a dramatic increase in energy.

If natural sunlight isn't an option for you, you can also purchase a high potency vitamin D3 and fish oil supplement to ensure that you receive a minimum of 2000 IU per day.

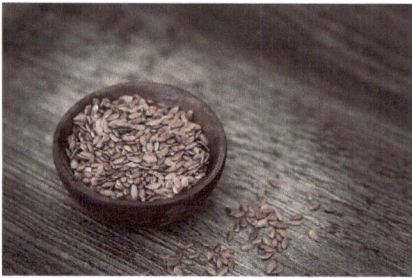

Flaxseeds are rich in plant omega-3s and help to produce a hormone-like substance which is called prostaglandins. This in turn helps to stimulate thyroid hormone production which helps to prevent and treat hypothyroidism.

8-Cellulite

This is a very well-known problem that millions of women (and some men) around the world suffer with. Cellulite basically describes normal fat beneath the skin which appears bumpy due to pushing against connective tissue. Although not a serious problem, it is certainly not desired and can be cosmetically unpleasant.

Each year, billions of dollars are spent for reducing the appearance of cellulite. Treatment options include cellulite reduction creams and surgical invasive and non-invasive procedures. Fortunately, there are more practical and affordable options available which need to be sought out and practiced regularly in order to remove cellulite for good!

It's estimated that 85% of women suffer from cellulite in the United States. It can affect women of all ages, shapes, and sizes which means that essentially anyone can have it. The most common areas of the body that are affected include the buttocks, thighs, back of legs, hips, and stomach.

What causes Cellulite?

There are many factors that can lead to the development of cellulite. The most common causes include hormonal changes as well as toxic buildup of chemicals in the fat cells. In addition, cellulite can be caused by an unhealthy diet, dehydration, poor circulation, and a sedentary lifestyle.

So what are some natural home remedies you can use to treat this embarrassing condition?

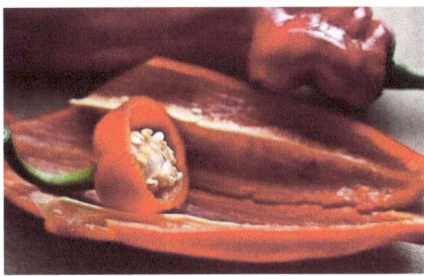

Cayenne pepper. There is very little that this amazing spice cannot do. It can absolutely help with weight loss and cellulite since it helps to increase circulation and blood flow. In addition, it is well known for being a strong detoxifier as well.

How to take:

You can easily incorporate 1 teaspoon of cayenne pepper in your cooking twice a day or more. Or you can prepare this drink:

- Add 1 tsp cayenne pepper
- 1 tsp of finely grated ginger
- Juice from 1 lemon
- 1 cup of warm water

Mix ingredients together and drink twice daily. This can be used for as long as you wish or until cellulite begins to disappear. Keep in mind that this needs to be incorporated with a healthy diet to help maximize your results.

What else?

Apple cider vinegar. Yes, again. This stuff really is the cure to everything isn't it? Apple cider vinegar contains essential minerals which help in detoxifying the body and removing excess fluid retention. This in turn helps to reduce the appearance of cellulite and if used for long enough, will help to remove it all together!

This remedy can be used both internally and externally. For external use, mix equal parts of apple cider vinegar and water and rub on the affected area. Wrap area in plastic wrap and place a warm compress on top (towel works best) before you take a shower. For internal use, mix 2 tbsp. of apple cider vinegar in a glass of water and drink before each meal. This can be done 3 times per day and can be repeated for as long as you'd like or until symptoms begin to subside.

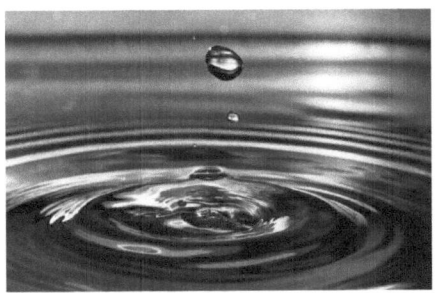

Water, water, water. This one seems like a no-brainer but many people do not associate being adequately hydrated with cellulite reduction. The truth is, water DOES help in reducing the appearance of cellulite by giving skin a healthy glow and smoothing the surface. In addition, since it helps with detoxification as well, you can maximize your results by making sure to drink at least 8 glasses per day.

9-Multiple Sclerosis

Multiple Sclerosis (MS) is an erratic and often debilitating disease that affects the central nervous system disrupting the natural flow of information between the brain and the body. MS is classified as an auto-immune disorder in which the immune system mistakenly turns on the body and begins to attack the cells including the myelin sheath—the insulation material surrounding nerve fibers. As time passes, this insulation gets damaged and can negatively impact the communication process between the brain, nerves, and other parts of the body.

Symptoms associated with this disease can vary dramatically from person to person however, the most common include; numbness, loss of vision, tremors or shaking, vertigo, muscle weakness, depression, speech problems, fatigue, and cognitive problems.

Standard treatment for this devastating disease are even more distressing. Toxic pharmaceutical drugs and steroids are typically prescribed costing upwards of $30,000 a year on medication alone. What's alarming is that these drugs are not designed to cure MS but rather treat symptoms only and slow the overall progression of the disease. As usual, drugs fails to address the underlying issue at hand.

So what can we do right now to reverse this condition?

Ginger, Cayenne, Cinnamon, and Turmeric. What do all of these spices have in common? They are all potent anti-inflammatory foods which help to boost the immune system. Since inflammation is basically the a key factor in the development of neurodegeneration diseases such as multiple sclerosis, incorporating these spices in your everyday diet can be largely beneficial in the long run as they will help to alkalize the body.

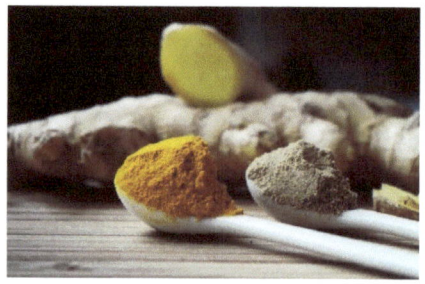

Turmeric in particular has been used to treat a variety of ailments including toothache, menstrual difficulties, jaundice, and even flatulence. This miracle spice can be consumed either fresh or in powdered form.

Here is a wonderful drink recipe to try using Turmeric

- 2 cups of almond or coconut milk

- 1 tsp of raw honey

- 1 tsp of Turmeric

- ½ tsp of Cinnamon

- ¼ tsp ginger powder or small piece of ginger (peeled)

1. Blend all ingredients and pour into small sauce pan

2. Cook for 5 minutes until hot (not boiling) and drink immediately

What else?

Calcium & Magnesium. Both are crucial elements for the stability and development of the myelin sheath. Calcium helps with communication between the body and brain via the nerve signals while magnesium assists in the muscle contraction and relaxation. Aside from trying to incorporate more foods with these 2 essential nutrients, a good idea would be to get a strong calcium and magnesium supplement.

An excellent way to absorb magnesium, is through the skin. This can be achieved by spraying magnesium directly on the skin. Symptoms have been said to decrease in as little as 2 weeks after starting this regimen. It should be noted thought that this can cause some skin irritation in the interim—a pretty small price to pay for big long term relief. You can purchase a pre-mixed spray or for half the price, you can make your own.

Here's how:

- ½ cup of Magnesium Chloride Flakes

- ½ cup of distilled water

- Glass Bowl
- Spray bottle

Directions:

1. Boil distilled water and pour into bowl
2. Add magnesium chloride flakes and stir until the flakes are completely dissolved
3. Let the mixture cool and then pour in spray bottle

This can then be sprayed on the body (legs, arms, and stomach), once or twice a day aiming for about 15 sprays per area. Leave on for about an hour prior to washing off.

What about the types of food to eat? Are there any that are better than others? The answer is yes!

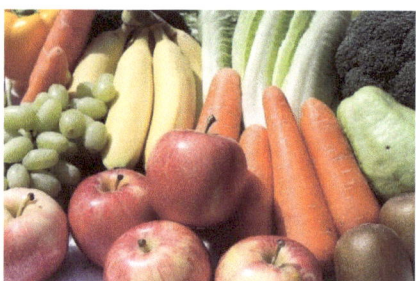

Fresh fruit and vegetables: Make sure to consume raw for maximum benefit. Seek out fruits and veggies that contain lecithin-a substance found in plants (and animal products) that helps to strength the nerves. Veggies that contain this ingredient include cabbage and bean sprouts. Of course, green veggies which are high in folic acid and B-vitamins are an excellent choice as well.

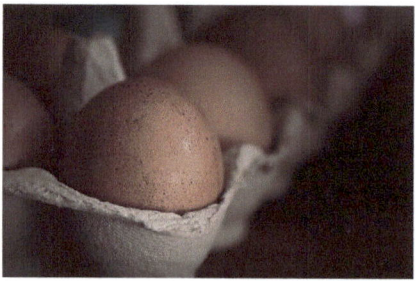

Eggs-surprise? Eggs are an incredible source of powerful nutrients and contain healthy fats which help support your brain and nervous system. For best results, aim to have at least 2 servings a day.

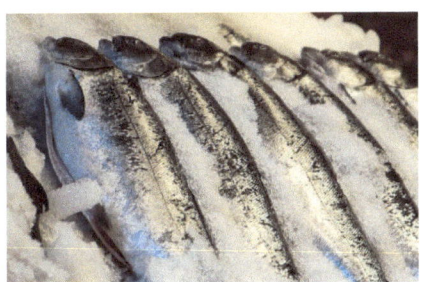

Fish: Cold water fish to be precise such as salmon, tuna, mackerel, herring, and my personal favorite, sardines. Aim for 3 servings per week if at all possible. Of course, if you cannot stomach fish—a supplement can be substituted.

Try and incorporate these foods/supplements into your diet and be prepared to see improvement. Of course, make sure to buy all organic when possible and try to incorporate exercise into your routine as well.

10-Urinary Tract Infection (UTI)

The urinary tract system is responsible for expelling waste and excess water from the body. It is comprised of the bladder, kidneys, ureters and the urethra. The kidneys are responsible for filtering and removing waste from the blood and forming urine which then travels down the ureters into the bladder until it is removed through the process of urination through the urethra.

Urinary tract infections have become widespread and common in our western countries. In fact, it ranks as second only to the common cold. The numbers of diagnosed cases are staggering and are said to be somewhere around 10 million per year. Needless to say, millions of dollars are spent yearly on treatments and doctors' visits and a great majority of patients are women. This is due to the biological structure of the urethra in women as it is shorter.

Symptoms of a urinary tract infection are not fun and can include (among many other symptoms) burning while urinating, frequent urge to urinate, and pain in the lower abdomen. If the problem isn't treated, the infection could spread to the kidneys leading to kidney damage. Symptoms of a kidney infection can be quiet severe and include fever, and pain in the lower abdomen and back. It's important to seek medical attention if you believe you have this infection.

Most people head to their doctors for treatment and are prescribed antibiotics. The problem with this however is that although they may be treating the symptoms in the short term, antibiotics rarely kill the microbes causing the UTI. In addition, they are killing the good bacteria in the digestive track which in turn, leads to the growth of bad bacteria. This can then lead to recurring infection within the urinary tract as well as release toxins into the bloodstream.

So what types of natural cures exist?

Cranberries. Sure, you've more than likely heard of this remedy but do you know why? Cranberries have been used to treat urinary tract infections for many years due to their high concentration of a substance called proanthocyanins. This helps to stop bacteria from clinging to the walls of the urinary tract. The urine is then able to essentially wash away the bacteria. In addition, cranberries are extremely high in a substance called D-Mannose. This has been studied for several years for its ability to attract bacteria helping it bind to it and then flushing it out of system during urination.

It was once recommended to simply eat cranberries or drink cranberry juice. After numerous studies however, this method has shown to be less effective than once thought. The reasoning behind this is that one must consume a large number of cranberries in order to achieve relief. Also, because most cranberry juice is high in sugar, it may have a reverse effect and cause bacteria to multiply further.

A more effective alternative is to take a cranberry supplement instead such as a D-Mannose supplement. This can have excellent results—and work quickly, since it contains a very concentrated amount of the compound. This supplement should be taken for a few days (1 tablet 4 times per day) until the UTI symptoms have cleared up.

Let's look at which foods can help:

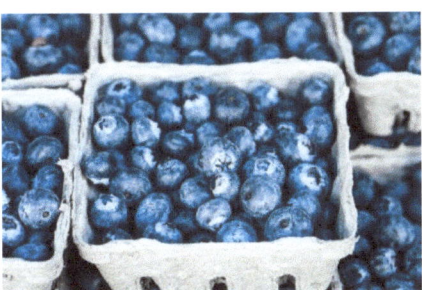

Blueberries: These amazing little gems are nature's perfect food. Rich in essential antioxidants, blueberries are known for optimizing human healthy by helping to combat free radicals that can wreak havoc on cellular structures and DNA. In addition, blueberries are an excellent natural remedy for UTI. In fact, they bear a striking resemblance to cranberries in that they contain the similar bacteria-inhibiting properties. Try and consume them raw and organic when possible.

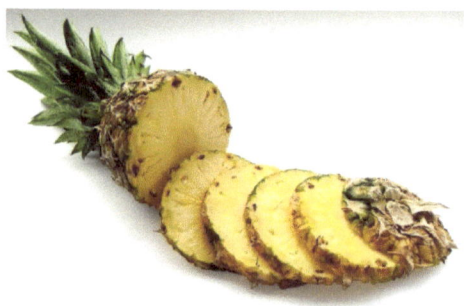

Pineapples. My personal favorite. They contain bromelain which is an enzyme that is known for being a fantastic cure for UTI. It is also rich in vitamin C which not only helps to strengthen the immune system, but can also keep the bladder running efficiently.

Last but not least...

Probiotics! You can take a supplement for this, or try eating fermented foods such as yogurt, kefir, kambucha, and sauerkraut. Probiotics help to balance out the good bacteria in your gut—and everyone knows that a healthy gut=healthy overall body! This includes healing the bacterial infection within the bladder.

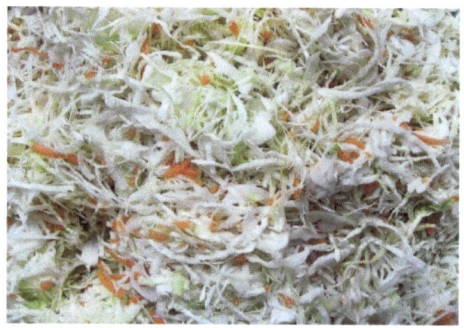

Here is a recipe for sauerkraut:

- 4 heads of shredded green or red cabbage
- ¼ cup of salt

1. Place cabbage in a mason jar and pound it to release the moisture making sure to sprinkle it with salt.
2. Keep the mixture below the top by about 1 inch to take expansion into account. You may need to add more in this step and make sure that the water extracted during the pounding process is enough to entire cover the cabbage. If not, mix 1 tbs of salt to 3 cups of water and add to jar.
3. Press the cabbage and keep under the brine putting pressure on the top using a weighted item such as a rock.
4. Place the jar in a warm area within the kitchen and allow it to ferment for 7-10 days. Keep it covered with a clean towel to keep bugs and dust out.
5. Make sure to remove any mold that forms at the surface and keep the cabbage immersed in the brine.
6. Once you are satisfied with the taste, place in refrigerator.

...And that's it! Easy peasy. This can be enjoyed alone or paired with your favorite foods (my favorite is brisket).

11-Constipation

This dreaded ailment affects the lives of millions of Americans each day. In a perfect world, one would have a bowel movement 3 times per day to ensure optimal colon health. However, bowel movement frequency varies among people. Some find themselves going 2 times a day while others only go about 3 times per week. This can be normal in and of itself. However, if one is experiencing uncomfortable bloating, and passing stool that is rock solid or large in size, it is highly likely that they're suffering from constipation. Anytime your stool is delayed by days or even over a week, and then accompanied by painful hard stool, natural relief should be sought out.

Being constipated means that the colon is not functioning optimally. This can cause unhealthy bacteria and parasites to grow and multiply. In addition, toxic liquids can then be recirculated into the body as they are not getting expelled properly causing a plethora of additional health problems.

So what causes constipation?

Although there are many causes of constipation, a poor diet is almost always the number one cause. This is because overly processed and refined foods are not digested as easily as natural healthy foods and therefore, are harder to eliminate. In addition, lack of fiber and an adequate consumption of water can both lead to constipation.

There are however many other causes for constipation. They include:

- Medical conditions such as IBS, cancer, MS, and hypothyroidism
- Stress and Anxiety
- Lack of physical activity
- Certain types of medication
- Over consumption of dairy products
- Artificial sweeteners

Let's take a look at some natural home remedies:

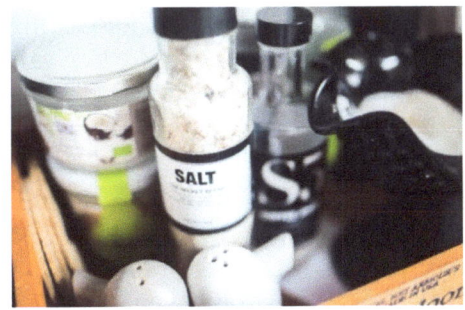

Salt Cleanse. What's great about salt is that it adds water into the bowel causing stools to soften up. This makes going to the bathroom a lot easier and more comfortable. Baking soda can be used as well as it has a similar effect. Both can be used together for a more severe case of constipation.

Directions for Salt cleanse

Mix 2-3 tsp of either salt or baking soda in cup of warm water and drink. This can be repeated every 4 hours until the bowels move. Keep in mind that frequently drinking fresh filtered water on a regular basis (at least 8 glasses per day) can help to naturally prevent constipation.

What else helps?

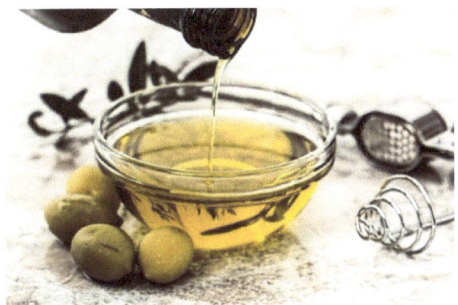

Olive oil. This is definitely a tried and true method of beating constipation. What's great about it is that most people have olive oil laying around in their pantry anyway and it's safe and natural to use—making it perfect for long-term use. Olive oil provides multiple benefits one of which is its ability to encourage the gallbladder to stimulate more bile which is a natural laxative.

What's more, its texture and consistency helps to lubricate the digestive system helping to move things through nicely. Rich in vitamins E and K and high in Omega 3 and 6 fatty acids, Olive oil can reinforce the health of your digestive track and when taken on a regular basis, can prevent constipation all together.

How to take?

Mix 1 tbsp. of extra virgin olive oil with 1 tsp of lemon juice and swallow. Repeat this once daily preferably before bed. Adding lemon can make taking the olive oil a little more bearable not to mention, lemon is also said to aid in constipation as well due to its high acidity. As stated earlier, this can be a long-term solution to prevent constipation but can also be used in the short term until symptoms are cleared. Remember to always buy extra virgin kind that is 100% olive oil.

Let's take a look at what else can help.

Black strap molasses. This dark, syrupy-like substance, provides a multitude of benefits and is rich in vitamins and minerals. What's more, it has a laxative effect in that it helps ensure regular bowel movements. In addition, it has high levels of magnesium and since constipation can arise due to a magnesium deficiency.

The best way to get relief is to mix 2 tbsp. of blackstrap molasses to ½ cup of warm water three times per day to help with constipation. Take preferably before bed.

12-Greying hair

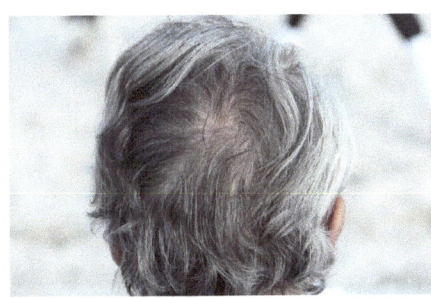

This is a problem we all face at some point in our lives and in most cases, there are no proven ways to treat or reverse grey hair especially when it is age related. However, premature greying of the hair can be treated and reversed. The best way to achieve this is to begin both internal and external treatments.

Since grey hair can be caused by a mineral deficiency, it's important to begin taking a mineral supplement. The best way to do this is by purchasing a good **colloidal mineral** supplement. Since colloidal minerals have all of the minerals the body needs, and is provided in a easy-to-absorb form, it makes it a great choice for fighting greys.

In addition to this, a good quality **colloidal copper** can be added to the regimen as well. This makes for an excellent topical external treatment as well—simply dab some of the liquid colloidal copper to the scalp and massage.

Although internal treatments are extremely important and to be used as the first step in reversing greys, external remedies can be utilized as well:

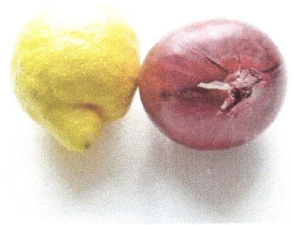

Lemon and onion juice. Ok, it doesn't sound very appealing, I know. But, this can be a very powerful remedy which has been used for several centuries in successfully curing grey hair—long before the inventions of hair dyes. Simply slice an onion and rub on scalp pressing firmly as you go to help release the juices. Follow up by squeezing some lemon all over and begin massaging. If you can get past the smell, go ahead and continue this treatment daily for best results.

13-Eczema

That "itch you can't scratch" feeling that eczema brings, is not only uncomfortable but can often times be painful as well. Not to mention, eczema can be cosmetically unappealing as severe cases can cause discolored or blistering of the skin. Eczema is the general term used to describe a non-contagious inflammation of the skin that results in dryness and redness in the skin as well as unbearable itchiness. Excessive scratching of the skin, can further aggravate the condition and lead to broken or bleeding skin.

There are varying types of eczema but the most common form is Atopic Eczema. This form is more common in children and can be triggered by a several factors including allergens, skin irritants, bacteria & viruses, temperature, food, and stress. Individuals living in urban areas and dry climates seem to be more prone to this condition and although children seem to be more susceptible, it can reappear during adult years as well.

Once the cause is identified and treated, symptoms of eczema can clear up on their own. It's important to take a look at the composition of the skin first before researching a solution. Our skin is comprised of the epidermis which is the outer layer and the dermis which is the second layer. The epidermis is composed of cells filled with fat and water; a healthy epidermis is rich in moisture because of these 2 elements.

The oils in the skin help with enhancing the skins ability to retain water. In individuals with eczema, this delicate balance is disrupted as the skin begins producing less fats than normal. This causes the gaps between cells to widen leading to an eventual loss of water and moisture from the dermis. This explains why certain types of soaps can make eczema worse by stripping away the lipids produced by the skin leading to dryness and cracked skin.

So what types of home remedies can work to correct the problem?

Coconut oil. We learned earlier that coconut oil has many wonderful benefits and can be used to treat conditions such as diabetes. It also has wonderful topical benefits as well and does an excellent job of penetrating the skin and filling out the space in between the cells and restoring moisture.

How to apply: rinse area with water and pat dry. Then, take a generous amount of coconut oil and rub into skin. This can be reapplied during the day as needed.

Let's look at what else works:

Make your own body-butter. It's much easier than it sounds, trust me! A good quality body butter can really be an effective treatment for soothing inflamed skin. This can be made using Shea butter, Coconut oil, Jojoba, and Beeswax.

Shea butter's amazing benefits come from its fatty acid compound which gives it an ability to repair and soften damaged skin. In addition, its properties help to reduce inflammation making it an excellent choice in fighting eczema. Beeswax is to be used simply for thickening this butter as well as protecting and softening the skin. Jojoba isn't an actual oil but a liquid wax and mimics the same oils found in our skin. Combined together with the amazing healing power of coconut oil, and you have yourself quite the treatment!

Here's how to use this remedy

Gather the following items:

- 2 tbsp. shea butter
- 2 tbsp. beeswax
- 6 tbsp. Coconut oil
- 4 tbsp. essential oil of your choice
- Glass jar

Directions:

Melt jojoba and beeswax in a double boiler. Stir in coconut oil until combined and lower the heat. Begin adding the shea butter stirring vigorously as it melts. When complete, pour in airtight jar and add a few drops of the essential oil. Allow mixture to cool and apply to affected areas as needed.

Let's look at a final remedy:

Cornstarch and oil. Yes, you probably have a canister of this in your pantry now...so go and get it. Cornstarch mixed with oil can be an excellent paste to help soothe the skin. Simply add equal parts cornstarch and oil of your choice (I recommend grapeseed or olive oil) and mix together until a spreadable paste forms. Be mindful that the paste is not too thick or thin. This can be left on the skin for 20-30 minutes and then rinsed with water.

14-Erectile Dysfunction & Impotence

Erectile dysfunction or impotence refers to the incapacity to achieve or sustain an erection sufficient enough for sexual intercourse. Although this can occur to men at any age, it is the most common among men who are over the age of 50.

Many people who suffer with this condition can feel down and alone in their struggles. Truth is however, erectile dysfunction is actually a quite common problem to have. In fact, it is estimated that more than half of the male population suffer from impotence (According to the Cleveland Clinic).

Often times, this problem goes untreated since most men find it difficult to open up and admit that they have trouble attaining and sustaining an erection. Many men even find it difficult to talk about it with their partner since sexual performance is such as strong indication of masculinity.

Let's start with addressing the causes:

Erectile dysfunction in and of itself, is not an actual disease but rather a symptom of another problem within your body. Some common causes include but are not limited to: diabetes, high cholesterol, prostate disease, hypertension, and depression. In addition to these possible causes, the two underlying factors associated with E.D. and also related to many of these aforementioned conditions are low testosterone and poor blood circulation. Coupling this with pharmaceutical drugs is a recipe for disaster as many of them can lead to additional problems down the line.

The good news however is that there are natural remedies that can treat E.D. easily and effectively. Let's take a look.

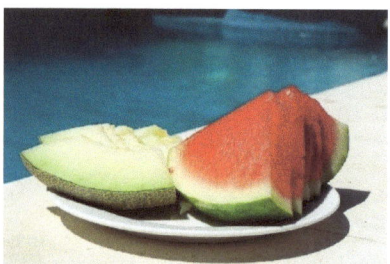

Watermelon. Your favorite summer fruit just got sweeter. Watermelon juice contains citrulline which is an amino acid that is said to improve blood flow to the penis. This one is simple, simply juice watermelon and drink the juice directly, or just eat it whole.

Cayenne Pepper & Garlic can be a powerful combination in treating E.D. This is because, cayenne pepper helps to increase circulation throughout the body and this includes the genital area. In addition, garlic helps with blood flow by dilating the blood vessels. Try incorporating them both into your cooking and if desired, try them in capsule form. These can be taken 3 times a day after each meal. Keep in mind that the cayenne pepper can aggravate the lining of stomach when taken without food.

Apple Cider Vinegar. You're not surprised, I'm sure. We've already taken a look at some of the wonderful benefits of this miracle food item. It can be beneficial to almost every ailment known to man and erectile dysfunction is no exception. The good news is that it goes to work within a couple of hours of consuming and usually only requires a couple of doses.

Although Apple Cider Vinegar doesn't treat E.D. directly, it helps to treat the underlying problems that are said to cause it such as the ones mentioned earlier. It also repairs blood vessels and nerve fibers within the penis and reduces pain and inflammation of the prostate gland. So give it a shot!

15-Dandruff

Dandruff is simply a chronic condition marked by flaking of the skin on the scalp. Not only is it common, but dandruff is rarely serious and isn't contagious at all. Aside from being an embarrassing problem, many people find it rather difficult to treat as most traditional methods aim at treating the symptoms only. It's important first to pinpoint the underlying causes of this condition.

Dandruff is the result of a dry scalp or a skin condition known as seborrheic dermatitis. In addition, other causes include eczema, psoriasis and more commonly, a yeast-like fungus called malassezia. This is a normal fungus which is present on normal, healthy scalps and only becomes a problem when it begins to grow excessively. This can cause the scalp to get irritated and begin shedding dead skin cells at a rapid rate.

Oil on the scalp then combines with the dead skin resulting in clumps known as "dandruff flakes". I know, it doesn't sound very appetizing. To make matters worse, individuals suffering with dandruff often times have very oily hair as well. The good news is that dandruff including severe cases, can be treated and controlled naturally.

Baking Soda. This one is up there with ACV as being extremely versatile and effective at treating a multitude of ailments including dandruff.

The best way to use this natural treatment for dandruff is to wet the hair and rub a handful of it vigorously into the scalp before washing off. Baking soda reduces the overactive fungi and leaves your hair soft and flake free. Although this method can dry the hair out at first, when used for a minimum of 2-weeks, successful results can be achieved as you begin to notice your scalp producing natural oils.

Olive Oil. This one happens to be my personal favorite as I always have a bottle or two of it in my kitchen! Olive oil is chock full of antioxidants and vitamins E and A which improve scalp/hair health by providing nourishment and reversing heat damage. What's more is that it contains antibacterial and anti-fungal properties which fight against the causes of dandruff.

Here's a method of olive oil application to try:

You'll need:

- ½ cup of olive oil
- 5 drops of essential oil of choice (I use lavender)
- 1 plastic bag or shower cap

1. Pour olive oil in a jar with the oil and shake well. Let sit for 12 hours in cool, dark place and shake again before use
2. Wet the hair and scalp and take 1 tbsp. of the oil in the palm of your hand and using fingertips, gently massage into scalp using a circular motion.
3. Place bag or shower cap over hair for at least 1 hour before shampooing

What else works?

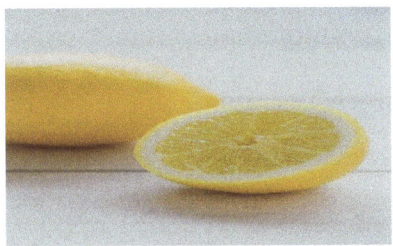

Lemon juice can be an excellent way to heal the scalp and treat dandruff. The acidity level of the lemon helps to balance the scalps pH level which in turn helps to keep dandruff at bay. Relief can be achieved by massaging 2 tbsp. of lemon juice into the scalp and rinsing with water. To maximize the results, try mixing the lemon juice with apple cider vinegar. The acetic acid helps to kill the fungus that causes dandruff.

How to apply remedy:

- Mix 4 tbsp. of ACV with 2 tbsp. of fresh lemon juice
- Apply all over scalp using fingers or cotton ball
- Repeat daily until dandruff disappears.

16-Migraine Headaches

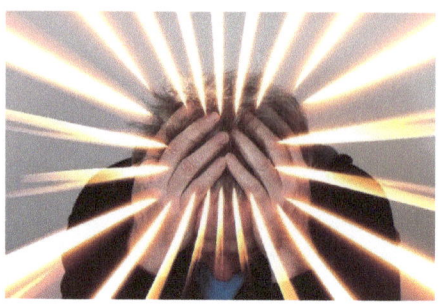

A migraine is best described as a recurrent, throbbing headache usually on one side of the head and frequently accompanied by extreme sensitivity to light and sound. A migraine can also cause more distressing symptoms such as nausea, vomiting, and visual disturbances (aura).

If you've ever suffered with a migraine, you know how painfully debilitating it can be. This is because migraines are said to involve neurological as well as vascular changes in the brain during an attack. For sufferers, there seems to be a genetic component that is responsible for the reduced threshold for pain including the hypersensitivity to stimuli. This leads to increased migraine pain caused by the inflammation in the blood vessels surrounding the brain.

Chronic stress may be one of the most common causes of migraines and other headaches as well. Because of this, many alternative treatments aim at reducing stress such as relaxation and biofeedback and are highly effective for many migraine sufferers. In addition, other methods for treatment include acupuncture, herbs, and massage all of which provide varying levels of helpfulness.

Let's look at some relief options:

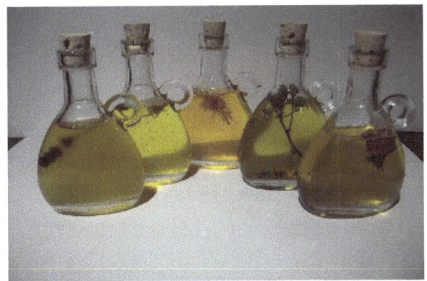

Essential Oils-*Lavender*, *peppermint*, and *basil* to be specific. These are all inexpensive and simple to use. Not to mention, they work great for migraine relief. Depending on your preference of oil (my personal favorite is peppermint), mix a few drops in 2 cups of boiling water. This can be used to breathe in the vapors with a towel over your head to help maximize the effect. In addition you can also apply the oil to the forehead and temples (dilute the peppermint oil prior to doing this). This remedy can be used 3 or more times per day to achieve relief.

Flaxseeds. Since migraines are essentially caused by inflammation, eating foods rich in Omega-3s can be helpful. Flaxseeds are rich in Omega-3s and can be enjoyed in several ways:

- Flaxseed oil-can be drizzled on salad or eaten by the spoon (refer to directions on bottle)
- Whole and ground flaxseeds can be added to smoothies and juices and sprinkled on cereal
- Ground flaxseeds can be added to bread mixture or soups

Last one:

Vicks Vaporub. In addition to being an excellent cough suppression, Vicks Vaporub is a wonderful cheap, home remedy for migraine headaches. Rub some Vicks onto the temples and forehead and then breathe in vapors. This can be repeated until the headache is gone!

17-Breast Cancer

This awful disease is responsible for the death of millions of women (and men) around the world yearly. It has caused so much paranoia and fear that many are opting for extreme precautionary measures such as mastectomies. This is an unfortunate fate that many are choosing for themselves regardless of the risks involved.

Because many people are unaware of the natural cures that exist, many are turning to their doctors and choosing harmful chemotherapy and radiation treatments. The problem with this is that these treatments actually promote more cancer in the long term as they destroy healthy cells and weaken the immune system further.

So where should a woman turn? They cannot count on their doctor to give them facts on natural treatments simply because their doctor does not know. Surely the pharmaceutical companies aren't planning on spilling the beans and risking billions of dollars' worth of medical treatments, no way.

Alternative treatments aren't only safer, but also backed up by several strong scientific literature. Let's begin looking at a few of them:

Vitamin D. This is only one of the several natural cures for breast cancer that have been said to work. It helps the body absorb calcium which is essential for maintaining bone health. In addition, Vitamin D helps to ensure that the immune system as well as the nervous system are healthy and functioning correctly.

Research suggests that Vitamin D may be effective at preventing breast cancer cells from forming. The best source of Vitamin D is the sun. This is why women and men are recommended to sunbathe for at least 30 minutes a day in order for their body to begin manufacturing the vitamin.

Here are some additional sources of Vitamin D to consider:

- Cod liver oil which is also rich in Vitamin D3, should be taken along with an additional vitamin D3 supplement.
- Salmon
- Herring

- Catfish
- Oysters
- Sardines
- Mackerel

What else can help cure breast cancer?

Baking Soda. Yes, we mention baking soda AGAIN. Simply because many swear by it for curing a wide variety of ailments including breast cancer. Best of all, it's cheap, and likely to be in your cabinet right now...go and get it!

Here's how to take it:

- 1 tsp. baking soda
- 2 tsp. grade B maple syrup or black strap molasses

Mix these two ingredients together on a spoon and take first thing in the morning. Make sure to stay hydrated by downing 1 full glass of water with this remedy. This can be continued for 4 weeks before resting. After resting for another 4 weeks, the protocol can be repeated.

Here's the final cure we'll look at:

Green Tea. We had mentioned Green Tea as a powerful remedy for diabetes. Did you know it is believed to be an effective treatment for breast cancer as well? No? Well now you know.

But what makes it great? Besides the fact that it contains extremely high levels of antioxidants known for neutralizing free radicals in the body, it also contains vitamin C and E. Also, natural chemicals contained in green tea not only prevent certain cancers from forming, they have even shown to reverse tumor growth. These remarkable benefits make green tea natures "wonder drug". Best of all, it's safe to drink every day!

18-Ovarian Cysts

Ovarian cysts are fluid-filled sacs within the ovaries that usually form during ovulation and dissolve after menstruation. They are extremely common in women of childbearing age and normally do not present any symptoms.

There are different types of ovarian cysts and most of them occur normally during the menstrual cycle making them functional. These types are normally benign and usually appear without any particular reason. There are however more serious types known as pathological cysts which can be either benign or cancerous.

Often times, women are not even aware that they have an ovarian cyst since they usually do not produce symptoms. However, in some cases, they can cause problems such as abdominal bloating, painful intercourse, menstrual irregularities, lower back and thigh pain, pressure in the rectum or bladder, nausea, and vomiting. More serious cases of ovarian cysts can even lead to infertility.

Depending on the type and size of the cyst, Doctor's may recommend the use of birth control pills or surgery to remove the ovaries and uterus. Although there are severe cases that may require these measures, the vast majority of cysts are functional and should only be addressed if they are presenting bothersome symptoms.

Ovarian cysts normally disappear on their own within a few short months. However, there are many natural remedies that can help relieve symptoms and even shrink the size of the cysts. Let's take a look:

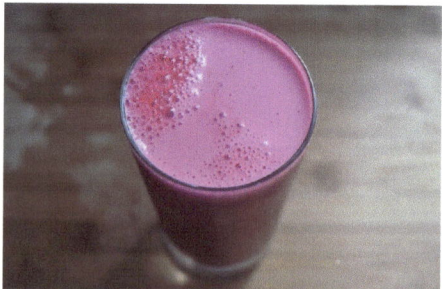

Beetroot juice is an excellent ovarian cyst remedy that many people have had huge success with. Beetroot contains betacyanin which is a compound that helps boost the liver's ability to flush toxins out of the body. In addition, beetroot is naturally alkaline which can help decrease acidity in the body and since disease cannot survive in an alkaline environment, your body will be able to heal itself.

Recipe to try

- 1 cup of freshly extracted beetroot juice
- 1 tbsp. aloe vera gel
- 1 tbsp. blackstrap molasses

Drink this once daily prior to eating breakfast and repeat until your symptoms have reduced.

Apple Cider Vinegar. Ok, no brainer right? This miracle substance can cure just about anything what makes this disease any different?

Since a potassium deficiency can contribute to the formation of ovarian cysts, it's important to get enough of this mineral in your diet. Because ACV contains high levels of potassium it can help to shrink and virtually dissolve ovarian cysts when consumed regularly. In addition, it can help control blood sugars which prevents the release of excess insulin by the pancreas. High levels of insulin can lead to other issues such as elevated testosterone which is the main source of irregular menstrual cycles, increase in body hair and acne in women.

How to take

What you'll need:

- 1 tbsp. ACV
- 1 glass water
- 1 tbsp. blackstrap molasses

Mix ingredients together and drink twice daily until cysts have cleared up. For best results, avoid taking on an empty stomach to avoid digestive issues.

Finally...

Castor Oil Pack. This remedy goes back many centuries as a powerful way to draw toxins out of the body by stimulating the circulatory and lymphatic system. What's more, when placed on the lower abdomen, it can help circulate fresh nutrient-rich blood to reach the ovaries and help reduce or dissolve the cyst. This method can be very effective but its use is not recommended during menstruation.

How to use

1. Start by pouring about 2 tbsp. of castor oil onto a large piece of flannel cloth making sure to soak the entire cloth.
2. Place saturated cloth onto the abdomen area and secure it with plastic wrap.
3. Then, lay back and place a towel on top of the abdomen along with a hot water bottle (over the towel).
4. Leave on for 30-60 minutes and then remove and wash area.
5. This process can be repeated a couple of times a week for a duration lasting at least 2 months.

19-Brittle Nails

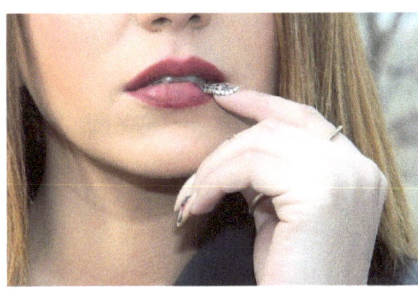

Everyone experiences brittle nails from time-to-time as they can be caused by numerous factors such as prolonged water exposure, aging, and through the long-term use of nail polish.

Weak, brittle nails chip fairly easily and many people describe them as cosmetically unappealing. Although the causes of brittle nails is normally benign, they can be caused by various diseases such as issues with the thyroid or lungs, psoriasis, alopecia areata, infections, and disorders of the endocrine system.

Other more common causes include dehydration, chemical exposure and nutritional deficiencies. Many times, a true cause cannot be pinpointed or could be due to multiple factors including the ones listed.

Nails that split or crack easily can cause some discomfort especially when the skin below the nail becomes exposed. When brittle nails are caused by nutritional deficiencies or an underlying medical problem, proper measures need to be taken to treat the condition first in order to experience long-term relief. There are however many natural home remedies that can help strengthen the nails regardless of the cause.

Let's take a look:

Sea Salt. This remedy is one that I hold dear to me as it has done wonders for my nails. Sea salt contains natural minerals that can help heal and strengthen brittle nails while adding some natural shine. In addition, it has an exfoliating effect which can help add softness to your cuticles.

How to use:

1. Mix 2 tbsp. sea salt in a small bowl of warm water.
2. Add two drops of essential oils of your choice (my favorite for this are frankincense and lemon).
3. Soak nails in the solution for up to 20 minutes.
4. Rinse off, and pat dry applying lotion shortly after.
5. This remedy is safe and can be repeated 3 times per week until positive results are achieved.

Let's look at the second remedy:

Lemon Juice can help in fortifying damaged nails and remove yellow stains on the nail surface leftover from nail polish. Olive oil can help enhance this remedy by providing moisture deep within the cuticles helping to strengthen nails. Mix the two together for optimal results.

Simply start by mixing 3 tbsp. olive oil and 1 tbsp. lemon juice in a small bowl. Heat the mixture just slightly and begin massaging into fingertips/nails. Leave on for 15 minutes and wash off. You should notice a significant difference after just a couple of treatments.

Tea Tree Oil. This was always my favorite go-to for various skin conditions such as acne due to its strong antiseptic properties. It is also useful for treating brittle nails especially when they are caused by fungal infections. In addition, it helps to treat discolored nails as well. This remedy is very simple to use and should be done daily until positive results have been achieved.

1. Begin by mixing ½ tsp. of olive oil or vitamin E oil with a few drops of the tea tree oil.
2. Rub mixture on nails while massaging for a few minutes.
3. Leave on for 20 minutes covering with plastic gloves to maximize the amount of penetration.
4. Rinse, pat dry, and follow up with lotion.

20-Irritable Bowel Syndrome (IBS)

According to the National Foundation for Functional Gastrointestinal Disorders, Irritable Bowel Syndrome (IBS) Affects between 25-45 million Americans per year with the vast majority of sufferers being women. Although the exact causes aren't known, disturbances within the nervous system, brain, and gut are thought to be linked to the disorder.

Experts have long believed that stress is the main culprit for IBS. However, it's less likely that stress actually causes IBS but rather can worsen or even trigger symptoms. This is due to the connection between the brain and gut. The underlying cause is often related to a poor-functioning digestive system which is worsened by a negative psychological state.

Unfortunately, millions of people suffer terribly and needlessly with this disorder and report a significantly diminished quality of life because of it. It's also important to note that IBS symptoms can mimic other more serious conditions. Because of this, it's important to have symptoms evaluated by a specialist prior to seeking treatments. Common IBS symptoms include:

- Abdominal pain and bloating
- Gas
- Constipation or diarrhea
- Nausea
- Fatigue
- Mucus in stool or when wiping
- Frequent urges to have a bowel movement

Standard medical treatments include anti-depressants, and anti-spasmodic drugs which do not address the underlying problems but rather treat the symptoms only. In the long run, these types of treatments can wreak havoc on gut by suppressing good bacteria causing, you guessed it, more intense symptoms.

Let's break this nasty cycle by looking at some natural remedies:

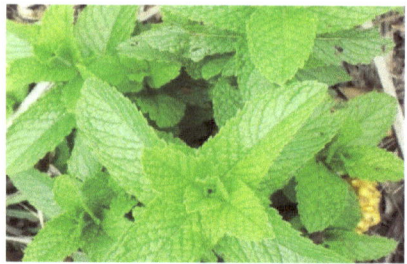

Peppermint oil. Peppermint is highly effective in treating IBS symptoms such as cramping, diarrhea, and bloating due to its menthol content. This has an antispasmodic effect within the digestive tract and can help food pass more easily through the stomach.

How to take:

- Add 4 drops of peppermint oil to 1/3 cup of warm water.
- Consume up to 4 times daily and continue until condition is improved.
- Peppermint tea can be also be used in the same frequency.

Let's see what else:

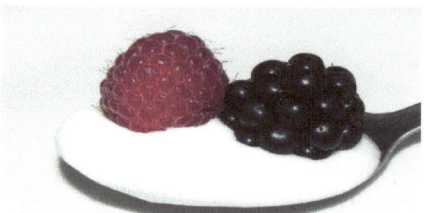

Yogurt containing live cultures has been known to reduce symptoms such as diarrhea in IBS sufferers. The friendly probiotic bacteria help to line the intestines creating a protective barrier that in turn flushes out toxins from the system. 3-4 servings of yogurt a day is best for maximum results and can be eaten by itself or added to smoothies. Try and limit sugar while doing this as sugar can have a reverse impact as bad bacteria within the gut will feed on it and multiply.

Final remedy:

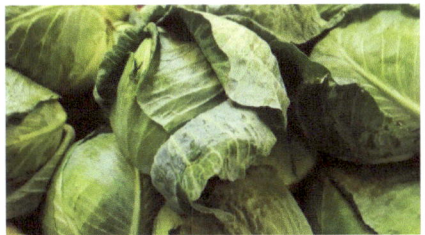

Cabbage juice. Yuck! I know! But stay with me here, it isn't as bad as it sounds. Raw cabbage contains sulfur and chlorine which cleanses the stomach including the mucus membranes and intestines. It also has a laxative effect which can help soften bowels and heal any constipation symptoms in IBS sufferers. Not to mention, it helps keep the body hydrated which is the key to optimal overall health.

Instructions on how to take:

- Cut a head of cabbage into tiny pieces.
- Run through a juicer or blender to make juice.
- Drink about a half of a cup up to 4 times per daily to help maximize results.

Conclusion:

I am so glad you took the time out of your day to read through these powerful home remedies! Many of them have been used for centuries and are proven to help treat some of the most stubborn health conditions. I myself have used many of them and know others who have utilized them as well with successful results!

Remember if you're already taking medication for any of these conditions, make sure to consult your physician about these remedies in order to make sure there are no drug interactions. It's important that you NEVER abruptly stop taking any medications prior to talking to your doctor.

Since natural remedies can take longer to work than traditional medicine, it's important to stay persistent towards your health goals and remain patient in the process. Although pharmaceutical drugs can get rid of symptoms fairly quickly, they hardly treat the underlying cause. The results of going the natural route, can be far more drastic and effective as they work to treat underlying problems rather than just masking the symptoms.

I wish you great health, happiness, and prosperity!

If you liked this book, please leave me a nice review and follow my Author page as I plan on releasing some more health-related content soon!

In the meantime, check out my healthy recipe eBooks now!

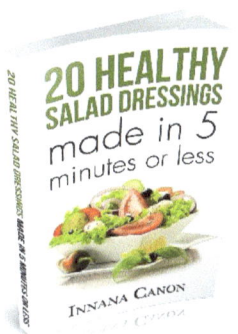 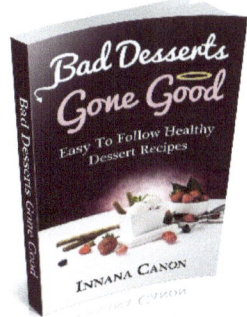